A Hero's Guide to Lifting Weights

Samuel Kennedy

DEDICATION

This book is dedicated in loving memory to my mom, Vonda Kennedy (1960-2016) who taught me early in life to value my health, and who continues to inspire me to be the kind of man she believed I could be.

CONTENTS

SAMUEL KENNEDY

INTRODUCTION

"I can do all things through Christ who strengthens me."
Philippians 4:13, New King James Version

What is a hero? History and Hollywood have both shown us a great many heroes of all shapes and sizes. From the rugged loner of Western lore to the colorful explorers who pushed back the boundaries of their world, to every individual who made a choice to do the right thing. That's what a hero is, in simplest terms: a hero is someone who does the right thing. Doing the right thing can be easy sometimes, but usually it isn't. Doing the right thing, putting others first, and stepping up to help someone in need all require commitment. That's why not everyone will be a hero. Anyone can, but not everyone will.

According to an old Jewish legend, there must always be at least 23 good people alive for the world to continue. Remember Noah and the Flood? An example of too few good people. Throughout history, a heroic few have often been all that stood between light and darkness. This world desperately needs heroes today. This is a global age, meaning a different set of problems face this generation than any generation before. Sadly to say, in many ways this generations seems least prepared for those challenges. Many are too absorbed in petty things to make difficult, meaningful decisions.

Becoming a hero requires commitment. It requires a passion to push through limitations and rise above the ordinary. Heroism grows in us from a million little choices that we make. Every time we do the right thing, our character grows. Do the wrong thing, compromise, and character is warped. Who we are is not built overnight; we build ourselves imperceptibly. Often, a person's character is formed accidentally, without purpose. A hero's is not. A person becomes a hero with intention and dedication. Each day, they give their all in the little things, and build the strength for bigger things.

Health is a part of everyone's life, but a hero looks at his or her physical wellbeing differently than others do. How do you view fitness? As a way to look good at the beach or a high school reunion? Or as a major key to achieving your full potential in life? If you think like a hero, you know that the stronger and healthier you are, the more you can accomplish. With the right training, you can live prepared for whatever life throws at you. I see so many people every day who are so out of shape they couldn't make it out of a burning building. They certainly can't help anyone else in trouble.

When I was a kid, I hardly seemed like hero material. In many ways I still don't. I was always the pale, skinny kid in school. Horribly shortsighted with no sense of balance or coordination, I was always the smallest, slowest, and weakest kid in gym class. But I was determined to change that. No one I knew exercised. There were no fitness magazines and no internet. My dad showed me some basic calisthenics and I started working out. Every day I ran, did pushups and situps, and dreamed of growing up big and strong. I've come a long way since then, and learned a lot. But I still have a long way to go.

Fitness, like heroism, is a lifelong commitment. I train constantly, learning new exercises and improving on old ones. Exercise is a way to conquer limitations. My progress in the gym reflects my progress in life. No matter what the world throws at me, I know I can adapt - just like my muscles adapt to heavier weights. Becoming a hero is a challenge I take seriously, so every day I push myself. I want to be strong for my family, for my community, and for my country. I train because I believe it would be selfish to take it easy and expect others to be strong for me.

This commitment to building strong heroes - heroes who possess both inner and outer strength - is the goal of my website, Building You Better.com. This idea grew out of a desire to help others find the hero in themselves, a hero strong enough to conquer any challenge. Exercise is essential to that journey. With Building You Better.com, I take what I've learned through years of hard training and package it in bite-sized pieces to help each reader reach their full potential. My goal is to cut through all the things that make fitness so complicated and bring you the straight facts so you can learn and grow.

Writing *A Hero's Guide to Lifting Weights* was merely an extension of that goal. It's true that everyone should master the bodyweight exercises first, but weight training is a crucial part of becoming stronger. Adding weights to your training is a great way to increase the intensity of a workout. It also places greater stress on the muscle than calisthenics, forcing it to adapt to a whole new level. Weight training has been proven to increase muscle density, as well as bone density, strengthening your entire body from the inside out. Besides all that, once you get used to it, lifting weights is just plain fun.

With this book, you will learn the basics of weight training. We'll take a close look at the different muscles and joints that provide movement, and at the best methods for training each body part. You'll learn about sets and reps, and how to train for strength, size, and definition. In the final section, I'll also provide a great workout routine, using the exercises you'll learn in this book, along with a few bodyweight exercises to round out your training. Everything you need to start your fitness journey.

If you believe that fitness is more than doing a few curls or a little bench pressing on the weekends, or if you're ready to move beyond calisthenics but you're not sure what's next, this book is for you. This is the book I wish I had read when I was a kid, and my fitness journey was just starting. Had I known then what I know now, I wouldn't have made many of the mistakes that I did. Hopefully, by providing you with this book, I can keep you from making those same mistakes. Strength and weight training are for everyone, and this book is for anyone who is ready to make the commitment and build themselves into a hero.

Having said all that, I have a question for you: Are you ready to begin?

PART ONE - THE MUSCLES

The human body is a wonderfully complex machine, almost infinitely adaptable. It can adjust to live in the Sahara, the Brazilian rainforest, the Canadian Rockies, and a million places and climates in between. Except for extreme situations, our body temperature remains the same in every climate. Our skin darkens to protect us from the sun's radiation in warmer regions. And our muscles become larger and denser as stress is placed on them. If you increase the workload on a man-made machine, the stress begins to tear it apart. But the body adapts to the amount of work it is asked to do.

Our muscular system is made up of approximately 700 muscles (experts still can't agree on an exact number), but most of them will never be discussed in a gym session. For practical purposes, we place the hundreds of muscles in the human body into a handful of muscle groups. Most of these groups are easily identified, though a few of the smaller ones can be confusing at first. Larger muscle groups include the back, chest, arms, abs, and legs. These groups can be divided into smaller muscles. For instance, the arms include the biceps, triceps, forearms, and shoulders; the legs are made up of the glutes, hamstrings, quads, and calves.

So, how many main muscle groups are there? It depends largely on how you count them, but I would say there are eight groups you want to focus on in the gym. I'll talk about each one below, and mention some exercises for each muscle. If you're unfamiliar with a particular exercise, don't worry: we'll be taking a look at the movements and exercises in Part 3.

Legs

The lower body may not seem as important as the show muscles of the upper body, but it is your foundation. The legs generate tremendous amounts of power during many exercises. Heavy leg exercises like squats can increase strength throughout the entire body, leading to a more powerful physique overall. Your legs make up half of your body, so don't neglect them.

Your lower body is home to several of your body's largest muscles. The glutes - generally known as your butt - are major players in lower body movements like the squat and in full-body movements like the deadlift. The quads are located on the front of the thigh, and are responsible for extending your leg, as you do in exercises like leg press or leg extension. Equally important, though less visible, are the hamstrings. Found on the back of your legs, the hamstrings do the opposite of the quads; they bend the leg, pulling the heel toward the glutes for exercises like leg curls or straight-leg deadlifts.

There's another muscle group on your lower body that some people train separately from their other lower body groups, while some people don't train this group at all. This group is the calves. Calves are responsible for extending the feet, and are used in every step that you take. This constant use - and the kinetic energy stored in your Achilles tendon - make the calves difficult to train, but unless you're a professional bodybuilder, big calves are not that much of an issue. Strong calves are important, but strong calves aren't necessarily big ones.

Back

The back is another area often neglected by novice bodybuilders. You can't see it when you look in the mirror, but it's just as important as the more visible muscles on the front. A strong back is essential for picking up heavy weights, as the back muscles pull the arms in toward the body. Any time you pull something, in any direction, your back is the main player.

Your back is divided into several big muscle groups. The erector muscles on either side of your spine start at your waist and moves all the way up to your skull. The main job of these muscles is to keep you upright when resistance starts to pull you down or forward. Moving up the back, we find the lats, which run from the shoulder to the middle of your back. Higher up is the trapezius and the rhomboids, both of which help in any kind of a rowing movement. In recognizing the different muscles of the back, it helps to remember that each muscle group is shaped sort of like a V and set into the group below it.

Now, I mentioned the trapezius already, but I think they need a little more explanation. When many people talk about the trapezius, they think of the upper traps: the muscles responsible for shrugging. But the trapezius is actually three muscle groups that cover roughly the top third of your back. The lower traps do a lot of the work in lifting weight upward, while also assisting the middle section of the traps in pulling from front to back. The last part - the upper lats - run from your neck to your shoulders, and pull weight straight up.

Chest

Like a lot of people - especially male weightlifters - I like to train chest. Wanting a big chest like Superman is the reason I originally started training, but I quickly learned there's more to strong pecs than just appearance. Just as the back is responsible for pulling weight toward you, the chest pushes it away. A strong chest will support you in any upper body pressing exercise.

From side to side, your chest divides evenly in half at the

centerline of your torso. Like the trapezius on the back, the pectorals are also divided into three sections from top to bottom: the clavicular head on the top, the sternal head in the middle, and the abdominal head on the bottom. Each is responsible for pressing your arms forward at a different angle. Forward at an upward angle for the upper chest, straight ahead for the middle, and forward and down for the lower chest. This allows us to train different areas of the chest merely by changing the angle of the exercise.

While the pectoralis major is the main focus in most people's chest training - and rightfully so - there are two other muscle groups that make a complete chest. First is the pec minor, which sits behind the pec major and helps with our breathing. The other is the serratus anterior. Though part of the chest, the serratus actually begins on your back, wraps around under your arm and connects to your ribs just below the chest. A well-developed serratus provides a full range of motion on pressing or pulling movements, and is also important for a balanced physique.

Core

When most people think of their core, they think of the superficial ab muscles on the front of the lower torso. While a good six-pack is part of the deal, your core is actually a system of muscles that wrap completely around your torso. These muscles are important for stabilizing your body and transferring power from your hips to your upper body for pushing or pulling.

The core's primary function is to protect and move the spine. This begins with the inner core, which includes the diaphragm and other muscles responsible for respiration. These muscles are built through heavy lifting and controlled breathing, particularly on exercises like squats or deadlifts. Moving to the outer core, we find more familiar muscles like the spinal erectors (the muscles of the lower back) and the abdominals (the six-pack). These muscles also protect and stabilize the spine, but they have a greater influence on movement - which is what makes situps effective for the outer abdominals.

Everyone wants to have a chiseled six-pack, and so many gym-goers make ab training a major priority. But in targeting the abdominals directly, they miss out on the strength benefits of indirect ab training. Let me explain. Since the core's primary function is to stabilize the spine, heavy movements that require more stabilization are often the best way to build a strong core. Take a look at professional fighters, or soldiers, or firemen. There's no denying that these individuals have powerful core muscles. Yet many of them don't have a clear six-pack. For them, performance comes before aesthetics.

Shoulders

While we're talking about performance versus aesthetics, there's another muscle group that looks great and is vital to upper body strength. I like to think of the shoulder girdle as the keystone of a strong physique. If you share my interest in old architecture, you know that a keystone is a large block placed in an archway. A keystone can support incredible weights, and that's exactly what well-developed shoulders do as well.

The shoulder's main job is arm movement. Your shoulders move your arms up and down, from side to side, and even allow your arms to rotate. Arm rotation is the work of the rotator cuff, four interior muscles of the shoulder. The rotator cuff is a weakness for many lifters, myself included. Your deltoids are responsible for actual arm movement: the posterior delt moves the arm back, the anterior delt moves it forward, and the middle delt lifts the arm up and to the side. All three of the deltoid heads connect to the humerus, or upper arm bone.

Because it is responsible for so much movement, the shoulder is more vulnerable to injury than most joints. Most shoulder injuries are the result of a weak rotator cuff, so let's take a closer look at this part of the shoulder. The rotator cuff provides stability in the shoulder; it's also responsible for arm rotation, both internal and external. These three functions allow the arm to move freely, while still keeping the arm in its socket. Arm rotations prior to a shoulder session can do a lot to strengthen your rotator cuff and keep you safe in the gym.

Arms

The last muscle group we're going to talk about is the arms. This is a favorite area to train for both men and women in the gym. In many cases, arm training means endless reps of complicated isolation exercises, but like any other group, the arms need a balanced training approach to grow. To understand your arms better, we need to break them down into three subgroups.

The first group we'll look at is the biceps, located on the front of the upper arm bone, or humerus. The biceps brachii is a two-headed muscle responsible for closing the arm, pulling your forearm toward your shoulder. Any curl variation will build this muscle, but it's important not to do too much: a relatively small muscle, the biceps is easy to over-train. The biceps' antagonist (or opposite) is the triceps, a three-headed muscle on the back of the upper arm. While the biceps closes your arm, the triceps extends it. Though often overlooked, the triceps are just as important as the biceps for balanced arms.

The final area we want to look at is the forearms. The forearm is responsible for hand movement and grip. A strong grip is vital for controlling the weight during a lift. Many gym-goers struggle with their grip, particularly when they start lifting heavier weights. At this point, most will start using straps to help them support the lift. Others will decide to strengthen their forearms through exercises that directly target the forearms or through indirect forearm training. Indirect training means leaving the straps off and building your grip by holding onto the bar as gravity tries to tear it out of your hands.

. . .

This brief discussion isn't meant to provide an in-depth look at the human muscular system, or how our muscles interact with joints to create movement. But I hope I have provided you with a basic understanding of how our bodies work. I hope that understanding translates to safer, more effective workouts in the gym. With that being said, let's move on to the equipment you'll be using in your workouts.

PART 2 - THE WEIGHTS

There is a variety of equipment you can use on your journey to building your best self. When I made the transition from calisthenics to weight training, I was still a kid. I didn't have a gym membership or access to specialized equipment. But since my dad worked in the construction business, I did have access to a pile of building materials in the back yard. I built my first bench and barbell using landscape timbers and cinder blocks. It was a crude set-up, but effective. I spent that summer working out in the Louisiana sunshine trying to put some muscle on my 120-lb. physique.

My quest for bigger, better muscles is ongoing, but fortunately I can now use much better equipment. Gyms and fitness centers today are stocked from end to end with every piece of fitness equipment imaginable. But the fact of the matter is, you don't need every fancy workout machine or device that comes along. Knowing what equipment you need to reach your goals and understanding how that equipment works plays a big part in the success of your fitness journey. For new people getting started in the gym, choosing the right equipment to use in their workout is often the hardest part of developing their own effective exercise plan, simply because they don't know the benefits or the drawbacks.

Most equipment you find in the gym will fall into one of two main categories: machines and free weights. Each has its own pros and cons. With machines, the weight follows a fixed path, which means beginners can easily learn the motions and stay safe as they begin their training. But as a one-size-fits-all piece of equipment, weight machines aren't as versatile as free weights, and they don't challenge your body's stabilizer muscles - which means slower gains overall.

I'm not saying you shouldn't use machines; I use them myself in many of my workouts and so should you. Machines are great for isolating target muscles and they're also safer if you're training alone. But your fitness plan should always revolve around free weights, whatever your goals. Free weights are endlessly adaptable, which means your exercise arsenal can grow as you become more experienced. So what weights do we have to work with? Well, let's take a look.

Barbell

The barbell was developed in the 19th century, and has been one of the most popular tools for building strength and fitness ever since. Originally, barbells used hollow metal balls at either end that could be weighted with a heavy material like sand, stones, or shot. Over time, as weightlifting became more mainstream, commercial barbell manufacturing standardized. Today, there are six main types of barbell you can use in your training. But before we talk about the different types, let's discuss the anatomy of a barbell so you know what to look for if you decide to buy your own.

A barbell is divided into three sections. The largest part is the center, which is where you grip the bar during an exercise. Portions of the center are usually knurled to provide a better gripping surface. On each end of the bar is a loading area, where the weight plates sit. Between each loading area and the center is a collar, which keeps the plates from sliding into the center. Standard bars use a loading area diameter of one inch, and accommodate plates with 1-inch holes. Most other bars feature loading areas two inches thick, and use larger plates with 2-inch diameter holes.

Standard Bar: My first barbell came from Wal-Mart. The bar itself weighed ten pounds, and came with an additional 90 pounds in plates. Five feet in length and one inch in diameter, it's what we call a Standard Bar, or a 1 Inch Bar. A great option for beginners, it's light enough and inexpensive enough to start you training at home.

Olympic Bar: This was my second bar, and the bar you will find in most gyms. It is the reigning king of barbells, weighing in at 45 pounds. Length is seven feet. Olympic Bars are slightly thicker than Standard Bars, measuring 1.1 inch in diameter. Its size and the heavy weight it can handle make it a more advanced tool than a Standard Bar.

Training Bar: This barbell is essentially a shortened Olympic Bar, usually about four feet in length, though Training Bars vary more than other types. A typical weight for this type of bar without the plates would be about 25 pounds. Smaller, but still able to use Olympic plates, the Training Bar is a popular choice for beginners and young weightlifters.

EZ Bar: If you've never seen one before, the EZ Bar may seem a bit unusual. Shorter than a full-length Olympic Bar, this bar features two curved sections in the center portion. This gives the user more grip options, and allows you to isolate specific muscles during your exercise. The EZ Bar is also helpful for those with wrist issues.

Fixed Bar: Like the Training Bar and the EZ Bar, the Fixed Bar has a shorter overall length than a regular Olympic Bar. But unlike any of the bars already mentioned, this bar does not use removable plates. Plates of a fixed weight are permanently attached to either end. The only drawback with this bar is the need to buy a full set rather than just one bar.

Trap Bar: Technically, this one isn't a bar at all, but a hexagon with an Olympic loading area at each end. Two handles allow the user to stand inside the hexagon to perform exercises. As the name suggests, the bar is often used to work the traps with shrugs, but it can be used for other exercises as well.

These are the six types of barbell you are likely to encounter in the gym. There are a few more unusual specimens, such as the Yoke, Swiss, or Cambered Barbell, but they are considerably less common. Whether or not your gym will have them depends largely on the size of your gym, and to a lesser extent on the demographics of its customers. All but the very smallest gyms should have most if not all of the six bars discussed above.

Dumbbell

The dumbbell is closely related to the barbell. It shares the same physical features: a central bar, collars, and loading areas on each end. The difference between barbells and dumbbells lies in size. While a barbell may be anywhere from 4 to 7 feet in length, a dumbbell is considerably smaller. Meant to be held with only one hand, a dumbbell also uses much smaller plates than a full-sized barbell. While a barbell is a great way to build raw strength and power, using dumbbells forces your arms to operate independently of each other, which can prevent or remedy imbalances and promote symmetry.

Like a regular barbell, many dumbbells use removable plates that allow the user to adjust the weight depending on the exercise and their own strength. Other dumbbells have a fixed weight. For a home gym, fixed weight means buying a full set of dumbbells, or three pairs at the very least. Commercial gyms all use fixed weight dumbbells almost exclusively, but if you decide to train at home, a pair with adjustable weight will probably be a much better choice.

Kettlebell

Another useful fitness tool is the kettlebell. Though still new to many, the kettlebell's origins go back to the 1700s. Russian farmers used the kettlebell as a counter-weight to weigh their crops, but they found that it was an effective strength-building tool. It was subsequently integrated into the physical training of the Russian military and continues to be a great tool today. It has become increasingly popular in recent years with the rise of CrossFit and other "rugged" training styles.

The kettlebell itself has a far different shape than either of its siblings. While both the dumbbell and the barbell hold weight on each end, the kettlebell has only one weight, with the handle positioned above it. Perhaps the best comparison would be a cannonball with a luggage handle. It unique shape makes the kettlebell ideal for some unusual exercises, particularly quick power movements where a bar would be difficult to balance.

Benches and Racks

Before we finish talking about the equipment you can use to grow stronger and become the hero we all want to be, let's take a quick look at a couple of other things you'll need in order to get to work. One is a good, sturdy rack to hold your dumbbells and plates. How strong your rack needs to be depends on how much weight you plan on using. Even more important than a good weight rack, however, is a weight bench. You'll need a good bench to perform exercises ranging from the benchpress to the seated curl.

When buying a rack or a bench, it's important to find a reliable manufacturer, as equipment failure can result in serious injury. A good bench should feel sturdy, yet comfortable. If you do decide to build your own home gym, you'll want a bench that's versatile as well. If you go to a commercial gym, you'll find a few different bench styles. Some are flat, while others are adjustable for incline. For a home gym, the adjustable bench is the best choice.

. . .

There is no limit to the variety of equipment you'll find advertised as "the ultimate fitness tool". Some of these items are great helps, while others are ineffective or downright dangerous. In most cases, looking for a simpler alternative is the best and safest way to go. Trust the equipment - and the exercises - that have a proven track record for producing great results. Speaking of exercises, let's move on and examine a few great exercises that should be a part of every hero's weight training journey.

PART 3 - THE EXERCISES

There are an infinite number of exercises you can do with a good weight set. The only limit is your own imagination, or perhaps your willingness to try new things. Each training style has developed its own unique set of exercises, while basic exercises like the squat and bench-press reach across all styles. Trying to figure out what exercises work best for you can be challenging. Ask any ten gym-goers what the best exercise is, and you'll get at least ten different answers. That's because everyone is different, and what works great for one person may not be so great for someone else. Even a casual look at every exercise ever invented would be far beyond the scope of this project.

So let's simplify things by taking a look at just a few of the many options available for each muscle group. While each person will favor different exercises, there are some that seem to work great for everyone.

Legs

Squats: The squat is the king of lower-body exercises. It can be performed with bodyweight only, or with a pair of dumbbells, or a barbell resting on the shoulders. Begin with your feet hip-width apart and squat down until you are almost sitting on your heels, then stand back up. If you have mobility issues, simply lower your hips until they are parallel with your knees.

Sumo Deadlifts: While a traditional deadlift is primarily a back exercise, this variation is an incredible way to build lower body power. With the bar on the floor, step into position with your shins just touching the bar. Squat with a wide stance and grip the bar with roughly six to eight inches between your hands. Keeping your back straight, pull the bar up from the floor, straightening your legs and driving your hips forward.

Lunges: A terrific way to build balance and symmetry. This can be done at bodyweight, or add a pair of dumbbells or a barbell. Begin with your feet shoulder-width apart. Step one foot forward and lower your back knee to the floor, then stand pulling your front foot in. Repeat the motion, putting the opposite leg forward.

Back

Rows: Absolutely the best movement to build thickness and strength in your upper back. Holding a barbell or dumbbells, lean forward or support yourself on a bench with your face toward the floor. Begin with the weight extended below you, and draw it smoothly toward your chest. Hold for a moment at the top of the movement, then lower the weight and repeat.

Deadlifts: There are many variations to this exercise, but in its simplest form the deadlift is merely a matter of picking up a weight off the floor and standing up. Begin the movement by standing with your shins against the bar, feet shoulder-width apart. Grip the bar with your hands just outside your legs. Keeping your back straight, pull the bar upward and drive your hips forward until you are standing up straight.

Pullups: This is one of the best bodyweight exercises out there, and becomes even more challenging when you add weight with chains or a weight belt. It's also a relatively simple movement. Simply grip a secure overhead bar or other handhold and pull, lifting yourself upward until your chin is just above the bar. As you lower yourself back down, make sure your arms are fully extended before pulling back up.

Chest

Bench Press: Probably the most popular chest exercise, the bench press is a simple but effective muscle-builder and is most commonly done with a barbell. Lying on a weightlifting bench, lift the barbell from the rack and hold it at arms' length above your chest. Lower it in a controlled motion until it is just above your chest, then press back up. This exercise can also be performed with a pair of dumbbells, at any incline.

Chest Flyes: For a lot of people, this is the only type of flye, but I like to differentiate between it and the Rear Delt Flye. Like the bench press, the flye can be performed on a bench set to any angle. Begin by pressing a pair of dumbbells with a neutral grip (palms facing each other). Slowly lower the dumbbells to either side, fully stretching both sides of the chest. Pause, then raise the weights until they touch each other, and lower again.

Dumbbell Pullovers: This isn't strictly a chest exercise, but the pullover is too great to be left out. One of Arnold Schwarzenegger's favorite upper-body exercises, it is a great way to finish a chest or back workout. With your back resting on a flat bench, grip a dumbbell with both hands above your chest. Slowly lower the dumbbell behind your head, focusing on the stretch in your chest and lats. Pull it back up and repeat. Keep your hips lowered for the maximum stretch, and don't use too heavy of a weight.

Core

Situps: There's a reason this classic remains a staple in any well-rounded regimen. While the critics say that situps will hurt your spine, negative results are usually the result of poor form. I would never recommend crunches, in which the upper body is rolled into a ball, but proper situps - with the torso kept rigid - are a great, safe exercise. Just remember to use enough padding under your back and hips as you perform this exercise.

Planks: While situps are great for your exterior ab muscles (that six-pack you hear people raving about), the plank is a better exercise for all the deeper muscles of your core. Unlike the situp (which involves movement), the plank is a static exercise, meaning you hold one position for a set amount of time. Start in a pushup position, then bend your arms until you are resting on your forearms rather than your hands. Hold this position, keeping the entire body rigid, for as long as you can.

Leg Raises: Another great exercise for challenging your entire core, leg raises can be done lying on your back, hanging from a chinup bar, or even on an incline bench. The point of the exercise is simply to lift your legs out in front of you against gravity. Beginners may want to bend their knees and only lift to waist height, but as you get stronger, keep your legs straight and lift as high as possible.

Shoulders

Overhead Press: The most effective way to build shoulder strength is also the simplest. Some prefer the Rocky Press, or Military Press, or the Hammer Press, or any number of variations, but just getting the weight over your head is important. Use a barbell as it will allow you to lift more weight than dumbbells. Hold the weight at the shoulders, press it up, and then lower it slowly. The Overhead Press can be performed behind the neck or in front, sitting or standing.

Side Laterals: A great way to build the side delts and the upper traps, giving you that broad-shouldered look everyone loves, along with some serious lifting and carrying power. Stand at attention with a pair of dumbbells at your side. Keeping your back straight - but your elbows slightly bent - raise the dumbbells at your sides until parallel, then return to the starting position.

Arnold Press: This variation on the Overhead Press is a great way to fully exhaust your delts and finish a shoulder session. Begin with a pair of dumbbells held at your shoulders, with your palms facing in. Press one dumbbell upward. As you do, turn your wrist outward until your palm faces forward. Return to the starting position, then repeat the movement on the opposite side.

Arms

Curls: There are a million "tricks" for building your biceps, but none of them are more effective than basic curls. Curls can be done with a barbell, a pair of dumbbells, or a machine. Start with your arms fully lowered in front of you, holding the weight. Bending your arms at the elbow, use your biceps to pull the weight toward your chin. Be careful to keep the weight on your biceps and avoid pulling with your back.

Lying Triceps Press: Commonly referred to as a "skull-crusher" or "French press", this is an excellent movement to build thick, powerful triceps. Lay on a flat bench holding a barbell above your chest. Keeping your upper arms straight with your elbows pointing up, bend your elbows and lower the bar to your forehead, then press it back up.

Forearm Curls: While gripping and lifting heavy weights regularly may be enough for some people to get big, strong forearms, some of us have to go above and beyond the call of duty. The Forearm Curl is the best way to do that. It is performed much like a bicep curl, but with one difference: instead of bending at the elbow, bend at the wrist. This is a relatively short range of motion, so aim for high reps with a barbell or dumbbells.

. . .

As I said at the beginning of this section, there really is no limit to the exercises or variations you can do, at home or in the gym. Some people respond better to one type of training than another. Some can use the same routine for years, while others vary their training from week to week. The important thing is to find what works for you, and grow with that. Use this short list of tried and true exercises as a guideline in developing your training, but never be afraid to try something new - using wisdom and staying safe, of course. In the next section, we'll take all the exercises in this list, throw in a few extras, and put together our own weightlifting program. It's time to take what you've learned in the last three sections and put it to work.

PART 4 - THE PROGRAM

Now that you understand your muscles, the weightlifting equipment you'll need to use, and the exercises that will help you build your strongest self, let's take a look at how we can apply all that information. To do that effectively, there are a few more questions we need to answer. How much weight should you be lifting? How many sets of a particular exercise should you do in each workout? How many repetitions should you do in each set? Answers to those questions will vary from person to person, but I'm going to give you some information to help you make informed answers.

Deciding on the number of sets and reps requires a basic understanding of several fitness principles, as well as your own physical goals. Beginners will find that a lighter weight lifted for more reps has greater benefits and less risks, while more advanced lifters will enjoy the challenges - and the rewards - of heavier weights and fewer reps. More reps per set means you'll be able to perform fewer sets; less reps means more sets. Age, height, gender, and cardiovascular ability all affect how much work we can do in the gym. If you're a beginner, or you haven't trained in a little while, starting easy with lighter weights and higher reps can get you started and keep you safe.

As you become more experienced at lifting weights, you'll want to move up to heavier weights. Exactly how heavy you want to go and how much volume you should lift in each workout will depend on your own personal goals. Higher reps ranges, anywhere from 10-16 reps per set, are great for building hypertrophy and definition - classic bodybuilding stuff. Lower reps, like from 3-7 reps per set, are brutal strength-builders. The exact results of specific numbers will vary from one athlete to the next, and even from exercise to exercise, but the principles remain the same.

For the purpose of this book, our goal is to train like heroes. Heroes need to be strong, but that strength needs to be functional. If you can pick up one end of a truck, but you can't jog around the block, you won't be able to help someone when you need to. Because of that, the course I've designed for you uses progressively heavier weights to build strength and mobility. By starting off light and mastering form on our lifts, we'll give our bones, hearts, and lungs enough time to keep up, while also jump-starting growth in our muscles.

At the end of the program, we'll be lifting a lot of weight for fewer reps in order to boost raw strength and power. While the big lifts will be the main focus of this program, we'll also do plenty of secondary exercises to supplement the Big Three. These supplementary exercises will help you build a balanced, aesthetic physique, but this is about more than just appearance. These secondary exercises will help support the big lifts, allowing you to become even stronger. They're also very important for balance and mobility, building strength in the joints and ligaments. Do not neglect this aspect of your training.

One of the mistakes I made early in my training was to always train heavy. I lifted too much weight too soon. I bench-pressed twice my bodyweight before I was even twenty, and had some bad shoulder injuries for my trouble. My muscles were definitely strong; in fact, they were too strong for my bones. Those injuries forced me to go back to the beginning and learn some lessons over again. I still believe in training strong, I believe in lots of volume in a workout, but I've learned to take steps to make my workouts safer. I've put those precautions to work in developing this program.

The program is composed of four one-week modules. The exercises are the same for each week, but the number of sets and reps change. You can go through the entire program in four weeks, or you can repeat a week until you feel you've mastered it. Every week, you will do three weightlifting sessions, and I'll be doing them along with you. I've used this exact program before, and I will be using it many more times as I move forward in my training. If you commit to it, and match hard training with smart nutrition, you'll be able to see some great results from this program.

The three weightlifting workouts will consist of Legs and Shoulders for the first workout, Chest and Triceps for the second, and Back and Biceps third. Core training will be a part of every workout. Since each workout is built around one of the Big Three lifts, the intensity will be high throughout the program. I recommend taking a day off between each weight session to allow your muscles to recover. Remember, muscles aren't built in the gym; they're built outside the gym. The gym is simply where we tell our muscles how much growing they need to do.

Your days off won't be all relaxation, though. A hero shouldn't just be strong, he should be fit. So let's talk a little about cardio. You've probably heard that cardiovascular exercise is the best way to lose body fat. That is not true. Exercise intensity matched with sound nutrition is the best way to trim off unwanted weight. Cardiovascular exercise is just what it sounds like: a way to strengthen your heart, and your lungs as well. This will indirectly help you lose weight if you need to, by allowing you to work harder in the gym, but it won't knock off those extra pounds by itself.

In this program, you'll be doing cardio two or three times a week - on days when you're not lifting weights. With our cardio sessions, we want to build endurance. A hero goes further than anyone else, and that's what we're trying to achieve here. If you have a pool or have regular access to one, swimming is one of the best forms of cardio - in fact, one of the best forms of exercise - you can possibly do. Jogging, running, or bicycling are other great options. I recommend at least a half-hour per session, but you may need to do less or more depending on your fitness level.

The most important factor in your cardio is the intensity. No long, slow walks on the treadmill here. Studies have shown that steady-state cardio can actually harm your progress in the gym, lowering testosterone and hindering protein synthesis, which is your body's process for turning the protein you eat into muscle. On the other hand, more intense cardio styles like HIIT (High-Intensity Interval Training) promote fat loss, increase aerobic and anaerobic endurance, and actually stimulate more muscle growth. And though it may sound brutal, HIIT is actually not that hard. Simply alternate between a couple minutes of moderate jogging with 20-30 seconds of all-out sprinting. You'll love it.

One more thing about cardio. If you're naturally skinny (like I am) you may find it difficult to meet your caloric needs while weightlifting and doing regular cardio at the same time. With my metabolism, it is almost impossible to eat enough food in a day. Perhaps if I ever find a perfect solution to that problem, I'll write a cookbook. But the best solution I've found for now is to alternate between strength-building and endurance-building phases. In bodybuilding, this is called bulking and cutting, and is hardly a new concept. Most performance-centered athletes don't use this training method, but if it's hard for you to build muscle you might want to give it a try.

Finally, let's talk a little bit about nutrition. Since it's such a vast subject, and dietary requirements vary so much from person to person, I won't be going in-depth, but I would like to quickly look at the basics. The human body is a highly complex machine. Like any other machine, it needs fuel. That fuel comes in the form of calories and is derived from three sources: carbohydrates, fats, and proteins. We call these macronutrients. All foods contain at least one macronutrient, but some foods are better sources than others.

Fruits and vegetables, grains, and diary are all high in carbohydrates, and are excellent energy sources. Diary is also high in protein, as are meats, fish, and even some vegetables and grains. Proteins are the building blocks, not just for our muscles, but for every cell in our bodies. And then we have fats. Unhealthy fats like trans fats and saturated fats cause unhealthy weight gain, clogged arteries, and bad cholesterol. In contrast, healthy fats help fight cholesterol, protect your heart, and regulate your blood sugar. These healthy fats are found in foods like nuts, avocados, and fish.

You'll need to be eating enough of all three macronutrients in order to enjoy the full benefits of this program, or any training program for that matter. Rest and nutrition are as important to growth as exercise. In the next four weeks - or however long you decide to use this program - make getting enough sleep and eating the right foods a priority. Then, tackle these workouts, really push yourself, and I promise you will see some great results.

CONCLUSION

Thank you for taking the time to read this book; I genuinely hope you learned something useful from it. I never would have thought I'd be someone writing about fitness, and I certainly never thought anyone would take the time to read it, so thank you for proving me wrong. I believe strongly in heroes; I admire those who take a stand and do difficult things even if for no other reason than that it makes them a better person. Building strength takes time, but it all boils down to the one moment when you make the decision to begin. I'm glad you made that decision, and I'm glad I can offer you some help.

This book is accompanied by a workbook, with a four-week calendar and workout log. Every workout in this program is included, with sets and reps. All you have to do is fill in the blanks as you do each workout. You can use the log to hold yourself accountable, and to keep track of your progress as you go through the program. This workbook is available for download on my website. Tracking your progress is the best way to reach your goals. And I do want them to be your goals - not my goals, not your friend's goals, not that big, muscled guy at work's goals; your goals. Know first who you are, and then who you want to become.

Remember what I said about heroes. Our world desperately needs them right now. Heroes come in all shapes and sizes, but they share one main characteristic: they dedicate themselves to doing the right thing, even when it's hard. Especially when it's hard. Training is hard, I won't tell you it isn't. But I believe you can do it. Trust me, I'm the skinny kid who always failed in gym class. If I can train hard and get results, so can you.

For more fitness information, advice, and great workouts to continue your fitness journey, be sure to check out BuildingYouBetter.com, and don't forget to download your free workbook while you're there. Farewell, and happy lifting to you.

ABOUT THE AUTHOR

At 25 years old, Samuel Kennedy has been a fitness enthusiast for two decades. Inspired by heroes from Samson to Superman, and encouraged by a health-minded mom, he began learning calisthenics before entering kindergarten, and built his own yard gym when he was twelve. Always the skinny kid in school, Samuel has spent years building his muscles and becoming as strong as he could be. Along the way, he learned that strength and fitness are much harder to achieve – and to maintain – than one might think. Health can only be won through hard work and dedication, but Samuel believes that it is the key to a successful, fulfilled life. His mission is to inspire others to become fit, and to help their strength journey in any way he can. He believes that everyone can unlock their full potential, and that ordinary people can do extraordinary things – if they have the right tools.

www.ingramcontent.com/pod-product-compliance
Lightning Source LLC
Chambersburg PA
CBHW030550290526
45786CB00004B/1948